Copyright © 2022 by Monica Dimitrios

Table of Contents

INTERSTITIAL CYSTITIS

Interstitial cystitis is a chronic condition causing bladder pressure, bladder pain and sometimes pelvic pain. The pain ranges from mild discomfort to severe pain. The condition is a part of a spectrum of diseases known as painful bladder syndrome.

INTERSTITIAL CYSTITIS RECIPES

1. Best Brownies

Prep Time: 15 mins

Total Time: 45 mins

Servings: 16

Ingredients

- ½ cup butter
- 1 cup white sugar
- 2 eggs
- 1 teaspoon vanilla extract
- ⅓ cup unsweetened cocoa powder
- ½ cup all-purpose flour
- ¼ teaspoon salt
- ¼ teaspoon baking powder

Frosting:

- 3 tablespoons butter, softened
- 3 tablespoons unsweetened cocoa powder
- 1 tablespoon honey
- 1 teaspoon vanilla extract

- 1 cup confectioners' sugar

Directions

1. Preheat oven to 350 degrees F (175 degrees C). Grease and flour an 8-inch square pan.
2. In a large saucepan, melt 1/2 cup butter. Remove from heat, and stir in sugar, eggs, and 1 teaspoon vanilla. Beat in 1/3 cup cocoa, 1/2 cup flour, salt, and baking powder. Spread batter into prepared pan.
3. Bake in preheated oven for 25 to 30 minutes. Do not overcook.
4. Remove brownies from the oven, and make frosting. Combine 3 tablespoons softened butter, 3 tablespoons cocoa, honey, 1 teaspoon vanilla extract, and 1 cup confectioners' sugar. Stir until smooth.
5. Frost brownies while they are still warm.

2. Easy Pancakes

Prep Time: 5 mins

Total Time: 15 mins

Servings: 4

Ingredients

- 1 cup all-purpose flour
- 2 tablespoons white sugar
- 2 teaspoons baking powder
- 1 teaspoon salt
- 1 egg, beaten
- 1 cup milk
- 2 tablespoons vegetable oil

Directions

1. In a large bowl, mix flour, sugar, baking powder and salt. Make a well in the center, and pour in milk, egg and oil. Mix until smooth.
2. Heat a lightly oiled griddle or frying pan over medium high heat. Pour or scoop the batter onto

the griddle, using approximately 1/4 cup for each pancake. Brown on both sides and serve hot.

3. Slow Cooker Beef Bourguignon

Prep Time: 15 mins

Total Time: 6 hrs 45 mins

Servings: 6

Ingredients

- 3 tablespoons butter
- 3 tablespoons vegetable oil
- 2 medium onions, quartered
- 2 pounds beef stew meat
- 1 (750 milliliter) bottle red wine
- 6 carrots, chopped into large chunks
- 3 sprigs fresh thyme
- 2 large bay leaves
- salt and freshly ground black pepper to taste

Directions

1. Heat butter and oil in a large skillet over medium-high heat. Add beef stew meat and cook until browned, 5 to 8 minutes. Brown beef in batches if necessary, making sure to not overcrowd the pan,

otherwise the beef won't brown. Remove browned beef from the skillet and place in the slow cooker.

2. Add onion to the skillet. Cook and stir until softened and beginning to take some color, 3 to 5 minutes. Transfer onion to the slow cooker.

3. Place skillet back on medium-high heat and pour in half of the wine. Bring the wine to a simmer, scraping up any browned bits from the bottom of the pan. Remove from heat and carefully pour into the slow cooker along with the remaining wine. Add carrots, thyme, bay leaves, salt, and pepper.

4. Place the lid on the slow cooker and cook on Low for 6 to 8 hours.

Prep Time: 10 mins

Total Time: 45 mins

Servings: 4

Ingredients

- 4 boneless pork chops
- 4 teaspoons butter, softened
- 4 teaspoons mayonnaise
- 1 teaspoon seasoned salt
- 1 teaspoon garlic powder
- 1 teaspoon dried parsley
- 1 cup shredded sharp Cheddar cheese

Directions

1. Preheat the oven to 350 degrees F (180 degrees C).
2. Place pork chops in a baking pan. Spread 1 teaspoon of butter over each chop, then spread 1 teaspoon of mayonnaise on top of butter. Season each chop with seasoning salt, garlic powder, and

parsley. Sprinkle 1/4 cup cheese over the top of each chop.

3. Bake in the preheated oven until pork is slightly pink in the center, about 35 minutes. An instant-read thermometer inserted into the center should read at least 145 degrees F (63 degrees C).

Prep Time: 15 mins

Total Time: 1 hr 30 mins

Servings: 24

Ingredients

- 2 cups all-purpose flour
- 1 ½ teaspoons ground cinnamon
- 1 teaspoon baking soda
- 1 teaspoon salt
- 1 cup unsalted butter, softened
- 1 cup white sugar
- 1 cup packed brown sugar
- 2 large eggs
- 1 teaspoon vanilla extract
- 3 cups quick cooking oats
- nonstick cooking spray with flour
- 2 tablespoons water
- 2 tablespoons white sugar, or as needed

Directions

1. Whisk flour, cinnamon, baking soda, and salt together in a medium bowl until well combined.

2. Beat butter, 1 cup white sugar, and brown sugar in a large bowl with an electric mixer until creamy, at least 2 to 3 minutes. Beat in eggs, one at a time, then mix in vanilla. Gradually mix in dry ingredients until well combined. Add oats and mix until thoroughly incorporated. Cover the bowl and chill dough in the refrigerator for at least 1 hour.

3. When ready to bake, preheat the oven to 375 degrees F (190 degrees C). Spray two cookie sheets with floured cooking spray. Place water in a small bowl and 2 tablespoons sugar in another small bowl.

4. Roll chilled dough into walnut-sized balls, and place 2 inches apart on the prepared cookie sheets. Dip a large fork in water, then in sugar, and use to flatten each cookie, rewetting and resugaring as necessary.

5. Bake in the preheated oven until light golden brown around the edges and centers are nearly set, 8 to 10 minutes, switching racks halfway through. Allow cookies to cool on baking sheet for 5 minutes before transferring to a wire rack to cool completely.

6. Jamie's Sweet and Easy Corn on the Cob

Prep Time: 5 mins

Total Time: 15 mins

Servings: 6

Ingredients

- 2 tablespoons white sugar
- 1 tablespoon lemon juice
- 6 ears corn on the cob, husks and silk removed

Directions

1. Fill a large pot about 3/4 full of water and bring to a boil. Stir in sugar and lemon juice, dissolving the sugar. Gently place ears of corn into boiling water, cover the pot, turn off the heat, and let the corn cook in the hot water until tender, about 10 minutes.

7. Classic Peanut Butter Cookies

Prep Time: 15 mins

Total Time: 1 hr 25 mins

Servings: 24

Ingredients

- 1 cup unsalted butter
- 1 cup crunchy peanut butter
- 1 cup white sugar
- 1 cup packed brown sugar
- 2 large eggs eggs
- 2 ½ cups all-purpose flour
- 1 teaspoon baking powder
- ½ teaspoon salt
- 1 ½ teaspoons baking soda

Directions

1. Cream butter, peanut butter, and sugars together in a bowl; beat in eggs.

2. In a separate bowl, sift flour, baking powder, baking soda, and salt; stir into butter mixture. Put dough in refrigerator for 1 hour.

3. Roll dough into 1 inch balls and put on baking sheets. Flatten each ball with a fork, making a crisscross pattern.

4. Bake in a preheated 375 degrees F oven for about 10 minutes or until cookies begin to brown.

8. Joy's Easy Banana Bread

Prep Time: 15 mins

Total Time: 1 hr 15 mins

Servings: 10

Ingredients

- 3 ripe bananas, mashed
- 1 cup white sugar
- 1 egg
- ¼ cup melted butter
- 1 ½ cups all-purpose flour
- 1 teaspoon baking soda
- 1 teaspoon salt

Directions

1. Preheat oven to 325 degrees F (165 degrees C). Grease a 9x5-inch loaf pan.
2. Combine bananas, sugar, egg, and butter together in a bowl. Mix flour and baking soda together in a separate bowl; stir into banana mixture until

batter is just mixed. Stir salt into batter. Pour batter into the prepared loaf pan.

3. Bake in the preheated oven until a toothpick inserted in the center of the bread comes out clean, about 1 hour.

Prep Time: 15 mins

Total Time: 7 hrs 35 mins

Servings: 8

Ingredients

- 4 racks baby back pork ribs
- salt and ground black pepper to taste
- 1 small onion, sliced
- 1 cup kochujang (Korean hot sauce)
- ¼ cup white vinegar
- ¼ cup minced garlic
- 3 tablespoons sesame oil
- 2 tablespoons soy sauce
- 1 (1 1/2 inch) piece fresh ginger root, minced, or to taste
- 1 (1 1/2 inch) piece fresh ginger root, sliced, or to taste
- 1 (12 fluid ounce) bottle pilsner-style lager
- 1 ½ teaspoons toasted white sesame seeds
- 1 ½ teaspoons toasted black sesame seeds

Directions

1. Remove membrane from the back of ribs or score with a sharp knife. Place ribs in a shallow dish and season with salt and pepper.
2. Purée onion in a blender or food processor. Add kochujang, vinegar, garlic, sesame oil, soy sauce, and minced ginger to onion in the blender; purée into a sauce.
3. Rub 1/3 of the sauce generously over ribs. Reserve remaining sauce for later. Cover ribs with plastic wrap and refrigerate 5 hours to overnight.
4. Preheat the oven to 325 degrees F (165 degrees C).
5. Scatter sliced ginger root over the bottom of a roasting pan. Place ribs meat-side down on top of ginger slices and pour lager over ribs. Cover with a lid or aluminum foil.
6. Bake in the preheated oven until meat is loosened from ribs but not yet falling off the bone, 2 to 2 1/2 hours. Let cool for 5 to 10 minutes.
7. Preheat an outdoor grill to 400 degrees F (200 degrees C) and lightly oil the grate.

8. Cook ribs on the preheated grill until browned, about 6 minutes per side. Coat with 1/2 of the reserved sauce during the last 2 minutes of cooking each side. Garnish with white and black sesame seeds.

10. Mamaw's Chicken and Rice Casserole

Prep Time: 10 mins

Total Time: 1 hr 20 mins

Servings: 6

Ingredients

- 3 chicken breasts, cut into cubes
- 2 cups water
- 2 cups instant white rice
- 1 (10.75 ounce) can cream of chicken soup
- 1 (10.75 ounce) can cream of celery soup
- 1 (10.75 ounce) can cream of mushroom soup
- salt and ground black pepper to taste
- ½ cup butter, sliced into pats

Directions

1. Preheat oven to 400 degrees F (200 degrees C). Grease sides and bottom of a casserole dish.
2. Stir chicken, water, rice, cream of chicken soup, cream of celery soup, and cream of mushroom soup together in the prepared casserole dish;

season with salt and pepper. Arrange butter evenly over the top of the chicken mixture.

3. Bake in preheated oven until the rice is tender and the chicken is cooked through, 1 hour to 75 minutes. Cool 10 to 15 minutes before serving.

11. Fajita Seasoning

Prep Time: 5 mins

Total Time: 5 mins

Servings: 4

Ingredients

- 1 tablespoon cornstarch
- 2 teaspoons chili powder
- 1 teaspoon salt
- 1 teaspoon ground paprika
- 1 teaspoon white sugar
- ½ teaspoon onion powder
- ½ teaspoon garlic powder
- ½ teaspoon ground cumin
- ¼ teaspoon cayenne pepper

Directions

1. Stir cornstarch, chili powder, salt, paprika, sugar, onion powder, garlic powder, cumin, and cayenne pepper together in a small bowl.

2. Use immediately or store in an airtight container
   for later use.

12. Chicken and Broccoli Stir-Fry

Prep Time: 30 mins

Total Time: 1 hr 20 mins

Servings: 6

Ingredients

- 6 tablespoons soy sauce
- 3 tablespoons cornstarch, divided
- 4 large skinless, boneless chicken breasts, cut into thin strips
- 2 cups boiling water, or more as needed
- 1 ½ tablespoons instant chicken bouillon granules
- ½ teaspoon ground ginger, or more to taste
- ¼ cup canola oil, divided
- 2 tablespoons sesame oil, divided
- 4 cups fresh broccoli florets, or more to taste
- 1 medium red bell pepper, cut into thin strips
- ½ green bell pepper, cut into thin strips
- 1 medium onion, diced
- 2 tablespoons minced garlic
- ½ teaspoon crushed red pepper, or more to taste

- 1 cup toasted slivered almonds

Directions

1. Combine soy sauce and 1 tablespoon cornstarch in a glass bowl or zip-top bag. Add chicken; stir to coat. Remove all air from baggie before sealing, or cover the bowl. Refrigerate at least 30 minutes.

2. Combine boiling water and bouillon granules in another bowl, stir until dissolved. Add remaining cornstarch and ginger; stir to combine.

3. Heat half of the canola oil and 1 tablespoon sesame oil to 365 degrees F (185 degrees C) in an electric skillet or in a heavy skillet over medium-high heat. Add broccoli, bell peppers, onion, and garlic. Stir-fry until crisp-tender, 5 to 7 minutes. Remove from the skillet with a slotted spoon to a serving dish.

4. Heat remaining canola oil and sesame oil in same skillet to 365 degrees F (185 degrees C) or medium-high heat. Add chicken mixture and crushed red pepper. Stir-fry until chicken is no longer pink in the centers and juices run clear, 7 to 10 minutes. Return vegetables to the skillet.

Add bouillon mixture. Stir until thickened. Stir in
optional almonds.

13. Mom's Peach Crisp

Prep Time:15 mins

Total Time: 45 mins

Servings: 8

Ingredients

- 4 cups sliced fresh peaches
- ½ cup all-purpose flour
- ½ cup brown sugar
- ½ cup cold butter
- 1 teaspoon ground cinnamon
- ¼ teaspoon salt
- 1 cup rolled oats

Directions

1. Preheat oven to 350 degrees F (175 degrees C).
2. Arrange sliced peaches evenly in an 8x8-inch baking dish.
3. Mix flour, brown sugar, butter, cinnamon, and salt in a bowl using a pastry cutter until crumbly.

Fold oats into flour mixture; sprinkle mixture evenly over peaches, pressing down lightly.

4. Bake in the preheated oven until crispy and golden brown on top, about 30 minutes.

14. Microwave Baked Potato

Prep Time: 1 min

Total Time: 12 mins

Servings: 1

Ingredients

- 1 large russet potato
- salt and ground black pepper to taste
- 1 tablespoon butter
- 2 tablespoons shredded Cheddar cheese
- 1 tablespoon sour cream

Directions

1. Scrub potato and prick with a fork. Place on a microwave-safe plate.
2. Microwave on full power for 5 minutes. Turn potato over, and microwave until soft, about 5 more minutes.
3. Remove potato from the microwave, and cut in half lengthwise. Season with salt and pepper and mash up the inside a little with a fork.

4. Add butter and Cheddar cheese. Microwave until melted, about 1 more minute.

5. Top with sour cream, and serve.

15. Southern Skillet Dinner

Prep Time: 10 mins

Total Time: 25 mins

Servings: 6

Ingredients

- 2 pounds ground beef
- 3 (15 ounce) cans sliced potatoes, drained
- 2 (10.5 ounce) cans cream of mushroom soup
- 1 (10 ounce) can whole kernel corn, drained
- 1 (10 ounce) can peas, drained
- salt and pepper to taste

Directions

1. Brown beef in a large skillet over medium heat. Drain fat, and return skillet to stove. Stir in potatoes, cream of mushroom soup, corn, and peas. Sprinkle with salt and pepper. Cover, and simmer over low heat for 10 to 15 minutes.

16. Edible Cookie Dough

Prep Time: 30 mins

Total Time: 40 mins

Servings: 4

Ingredients

- ¾ cup packed brown sugar
- ½ cup butter
- 1 teaspoon vanilla extract
- ½ teaspoon salt
- 1 cup all-purpose flour
- 2 tablespoons milk
- ½ cup milk chocolate chips
- ½ cup mini chocolate chips

Directions

1. Combine brown sugar and butter in a large bowl; beat with an electric mixer until creamy. Beat in vanilla extract and salt. Add flour; mix until a crumbly dough forms. Mix in milk. Fold in milk chocolate chips and mini chocolate chips.

17. Spaghetti Sauce with Ground Beef

Prep Time: 10 mins

Total Time: 1 hr 15 mins

Servings: 8

Ingredients

- 1 pound ground beef
- 1 medium onion, chopped
- 4 cloves garlic, minced
- 1 small green bell pepper, diced
- 1 (28 ounce) can diced tomatoes
- 1 (16 ounce) can tomato sauce
- 1 (6 ounce) can tomato paste
- 2 teaspoons dried oregano
- 2 teaspoons dried basil
- 1 teaspoon salt
- ½ teaspoon ground black pepper

Directions

1. Combine ground beef, onion, garlic, and green pepper in a large saucepan over medium-high heat. Cook and stir until meat is browned and crumbly and vegetables are tender, 5 to 7 minutes. Drain grease.
2. Stir diced tomatoes, tomato sauce, and tomato paste into the pan. Season with oregano, basil, salt, and pepper. Simmer spaghetti sauce for 1 hour, stirring occasionally.

18. Quick Tartar Sauce

Prep Time: 5 mins

Total Time: 5 mins

Servings: 8

Ingredients

- 1 cup mayonnaise
- 2 teaspoons sweet pickle relish
- 1 teaspoon prepared yellow mustard
- 1 teaspoon lemon juice

Directions

1. Stir mayonnaise, relish, mustard, and lemon juice together in a bowl.

Prep Time: 30 mins

Total Time: 1 hr 20 mins

Servings: 12

Ingredients

- 10 cups all-purpose apples, peeled, cored and sliced
- 1 cup white sugar
- 1 tablespoon all-purpose flour
- 1 teaspoon ground cinnamon
- ½ cup water
- 1 cup quick-cooking oats
- 1 cup all-purpose flour
- 1 cup packed brown sugar
- ¼ teaspoon baking powder
- ¼ teaspoon baking soda
- ½ cup butter, melted

Directions

1. Preheat oven to 350 degrees F (175 degree C).

2. Place the sliced apples in a 9x13 inch pan. Mix the white sugar, 1 tablespoon flour and ground cinnamon together, and sprinkle over apples. Pour water evenly over all.

3. Combine the oats, 1 cup flour, brown sugar, baking powder, baking soda and melted butter together. Crumble evenly over the apple mixture.

4. Bake at 350 degrees F (175 degrees C) for about 45 minutes.

Prep Time: 20 mins

Total Time: 30 mins

Servings: 4

Ingredients

- 2 cups grated zucchini
- 2 eggs, beaten
- ½ cup all-purpose flour
- ½ cup grated Parmesan cheese
- ½ cup shredded mozzarella cheese
- ¼ cup chopped onion
- salt to taste
- 2 tablespoons vegetable oil

Directions

1. Combine zucchini, eggs, flour, Parmesan cheese, mozzarella cheese, onion, and salt in a medium bowl. Stir well enough to distribute ingredients evenly.
2. Heat oil in a skillet over medium-high heat.

3. Working in batches, scoop tablespoonfuls of
   zucchini mixture into hot oil and fry until golden
   brown, about 2 minutes per side.

21. Perfect Sushi Rice

Prep Time: 5 mins

Total Time: 25 mins

Servings: 15

Ingredients

- 2 cups uncooked glutinous white rice
- 3 cups water
- ½ cup rice vinegar
- 1 tablespoon vegetable oil
- ¼ cup white sugar
- 1 teaspoon salt

Directions

1. Rinse the rice in a strainer or colander under cold running water until the water runs clear.
2. Combine rice and water in a saucepan over medium-high heat and bring to a boil. Reduce heat to low, cover, and cook until rice is tender and all water has been absorbed, about 20 minutes. Remove from stove and set aside until cool enough to handle.

3. Meanwhile, combine rice vinegar, oil, sugar, and salt in a small saucepan over medium heat. Cook until the sugar has dissolved. Allow to cool, then stir into the cooked rice. While mixture will appear very wet at first, keep stirring and rice will dry as it cools.

22. Spicy Shrimp Fettuccine with Garlic and Tomatoes

Prep Time: 15 mins

Total Time: 40 mins

Servings: 2

Ingredients

- 4 ounces dry fettuccine pasta
- 4 tablespoons extra-virgin olive oil
- 1 onion, finely chopped
- 1 rib celery, chopped
- 3 cloves garlic, finely chopped
- 2 chile peppers, seeded and diced
- ¾ pound large uncooked shrimp
- 4 large tomatoes, chopped into small pieces
- 1 bunch fresh parsley, chopped
- 1 lemon, juiced
- ½ teaspoon white sugar
- sea salt and freshly ground pepper

Directions

1. Fill a large pot with lightly salted water and bring to a rolling boil. Cook fettuccine at a boil until tender yet firm to the bite, about 8 minutes.

2. Meanwhile, heat oil in a large skillet over medium heat. Add onion, celery, and garlic and cook until soft, 3 to 5 minutes. Stir in chile peppers and cook for 5 minutes.

3. Add shrimp and cook until opaque, about 3 minutes. Stir in tomatoes and parsley and cook for 5 minutes. Season with lemon juice and sugar and cook for 5 minutes. Season with salt and pepper.

4. Drain fettucine and toss with shrimp mixture.

23. Buttery Garlic Green Beans

Prep Time: 5 mins

Total Time: 15 mins

Servings: 4

Ingredients

- 1 pound fresh green beans, trimmed and snapped in half
- 3 tablespoons butter
- 3 cloves garlic, minced
- ⅛ teaspoon lemon-pepper seasoning, or more to taste
- salt to taste

Directions

1. Place green beans into a large skillet and cover with water; bring to a boil. Reduce heat to medium-low and simmer until beans just start to soften, 3 to 5 minutes. Drain and return to the skillet.

2. Add butter and stir until melted, 1 to 2 minutes.

3. Add garlic; cook until tender and fragrant, 1 to 2
   minutes.
4. Season with lemon-pepper seasoning and salt
   before serving.

24. Quick and Easy Pizza Crust

Prep Time: 10 mins

Total Time: 45 mins

Servings: 8

Ingredients

- 1 cup warm water (110 degrees F/45 degrees C)
- 1 (.25 ounce) package active dry yeast
- 1 teaspoon white sugar
- 2 ½ cups bread flour
- 2 tablespoons olive oil
- 1 teaspoon salt

Directions

1. Preheat oven to 450 degrees F (230 degrees C). Lightly grease a pizza pan.
2. Place warm water in a bowl; add yeast and sugar. Mix and let stand until creamy, about 10 minutes.
3. Add flour, oil, and salt to the yeast mixture; beat until smooth. You can do this by hand or use a stand mixer fitted with a dough hook to make it easier. Let rest for 5 minutes.

4. Turn dough out onto a lightly floured surface and pat or roll into a 12-inch circle. Transfer to the prepared pizza pan.
5. Spread crust with sauce and toppings of your choice.
6. Bake in the preheated oven until golden brown, 15 to 20 minutes. Remove from the oven and let cool for 5 minutes before serving.

Prep Time: 30 mins

Total Time: 1 hr 55 mins

Servings: 6

Ingredients

- 8 ounces rotini pasta
- 1 pound ground beef
- ½ pound bulk mild Italian sausage
- ¾ cup chopped onion
- ¼ cup chopped celery
- 1 clove garlic, minced
- 1 tablespoon minced green bell pepper
- salt and pepper to taste
- 1 (14.4 ounce) can diced tomatoes
- 1 (15 ounce) can tomato sauce
- 2 cups shredded Italian cheese blend
- 1 ½ cups shredded sharp Cheddar cheese

Directions

1. Preheat oven to 350 degrees F (175 degrees C).

2. Bring a large pot of lightly salted water to a boil. Add pasta and cook until just al dente, 6 to 8 minutes; drain. Run cold water over the pasta to stop pasta from cooking further. Set aside.

3. Meanwhile, cook the ground beef and sausage until completely browned and crumbled, 7 to 10 minutes. Mix in the onion, celery, garlic, and pepper; continue to cook and stir another 5 minutes. Season with salt and pepper. Remove from heat and stir in tomatoes and tomato sauce. Allow to cool five minutes.

4. Lightly grease a large casserole dish. Spread the pasta over the bottom of the dish. Sprinkle the Italian cheese blend over the pasta. Pour the meat mixture over the pasta and cheese. Cover dish with heavy aluminum foil. Bake in preheated oven for 45 minutes; remove foil and sprinkle Cheddar cheese evenly over the casserole. Continue baking until Cheddar cheese has melted, about 5 minutes. Rest for 10 minutes before serving.

Prep Time: 30 mins

Total Time: 1 hr 30 mins

Servings: 8

Ingredients

- 8 small Granny Smith apples, or as needed
- ½ cup unsalted butter
- 3 tablespoons all-purpose flour
- ½ cup white sugar
- ½ cup packed brown sugar
- ¼ cup water
- 1 (9 inch) double-crust pie pastry, thawed

Directions

1. Peel and core apples, then thinly slice. Set aside.
2. Preheat the oven to 425 degrees F (220 degrees C).
3. Melt butter in a saucepan over medium heat. Add flour and stir to form a paste; cook until fragrant, about 1 to 2 minutes. Add bothn sugars and

water; bring to a boil. Reduce the heat to low and simmer for 3 to 5 minutes. Remove from the heat.

4. Press one pastry into the bottom and up the sides of a 9-inch pie pan. Roll out remaining pastry so it will overhang the pie by about 1/2 inch. Cut pastry into eight 1-inch strips.

5. Place sliced apples in the bottom crust, forming a slight mound.

6. Lay four strips vertically and evenly spaced over top of the filled pie, using longer strips in the center and shorter strips at the edges.

7. Fold the first and third strips all the way back so they're almost falling off the pie. Lay one of the unused strips perpendicular over the second and forth strips, then unfold the first and third strips back into their original position.

8. Fold the second and forth vertical strips back. Lay one of the three unused strips perpendicular over top. Unfold the first and third strips back into their original position.

9. Repeat Steps 7 and 8 to weave in the last two strips of pastry. Fold and trim excess dough at the edges as necessary, and pinch to secure.

10. Slowly and gently pour the sugar-butter mixture over the crust, making sure it seeps down through the lattice and over the sliced apples. Brush some over the top of the lattice, but make sure it doesn't run off the sides.

11. Bake in the preheated oven for 15 minutes. Reduce the temperature to 350 degrees F (175 degrees C) and continue baking until apples are soft, 35 to 45 minutes.

Prep Time: 15 mins

Total Time: 40 mins

Servings: 6

Ingredients

- ½ cup cream cheese
- ½ cup shredded sharp Cheddar cheese
- 12 jalapeno peppers, halved lengthwise, seeds and membranes removed
- 12 slices bacon

Directions

1. Preheat oven to 400 degrees F (200 degrees C). Line a baking sheet with aluminum foil.
2. Mix cream cheese and Cheddar cheese together in a bowl until evenly blended. Fill each jalapeno half with the cheese mixture. Put halves back together and wrap each stuffed pepper with a slice of bacon. Arrange bacon-wrapped peppers on the prepared baking sheet.

3. Bake in the preheated oven until bacon is crispy,
    25 to 35 minutes.

Prep Time: 10 mins

Total Time: 50 mins

Servings: 60

Ingredients

- 10 pounds fresh small beets, stems removed
- 2 cups white sugar
- 1 tablespoon pickling salt
- 1 quart white vinegar
- ¼ cup whole cloves, or as needed

Directions

1. Place beets in a large stockpot with water to cover. Bring to a boil, and cook until tender, about 15 minutes.
2. Meanwhile, inspect 10 pint-sized jars for cracks and rings for rust, discarding any defective ones. Immerse in simmering water until beets are ready. Wash new, unused lids and rings in warm soapy water.

3. Drain beets, reserving 2 cups of beet water. When beets are cool enough to handle, peel and discard skins.

4. Fill each sterilized jar with beets. Evenly divide cloves among the jars.

5. Combine sugar, 2 cups of beet water, vinegar, and pickling salt in a large saucepan; bring to a rapid boil.

6. Pour the hot brine over the beets in the jars, and seal the lids.

7. Place a rack in the bottom of a large stockpot and fill halfway with water. Bring to a boil over high heat, then carefully lower the jars into the pot using a holder. Leave a 2-inch space between the jars. Pour in more boiling water if necessary until the water level is at least 1 inch above the tops of the jars. Bring the water to a full boil, cover the pot, and process for 10 minutes.

29. Buffalo Chicken Wing Sauce

Total Time: 5 mins

Servings: 8

Ingredients

- ⅔ cup hot pepper sauce
- ½ cup cold unsalted butter
- 1 ½ tablespoons white vinegar
- ¼ teaspoon Worcestershire sauce
- ¼ teaspoon cayenne pepper
- ⅛ teaspoon garlic powder
- salt to tasteDirections

1. Combine hot sauce, butter, vinegar, Worcestershire sauce, cayenne, garlic powder, and salt in a pot over medium heat. Bring to a simmer while stirring with a whisk.
2. As soon as the liquid begins to bubble on the sides of the pot, remove from heat, stir with the whisk, and set aside for use.

Prep Time: 10 mins

Total Time: 40 mins

Servings: 8

Ingredients

- 1 pound ground beef
- 1 pinch salt and ground black pepper to taste
- 1 (10.75 ounce) can condensed cream of mushroom soup
- 2 cups shredded Cheddar cheese
- 1 (16 ounce) package frozen tater tots

Directions

3. Preheat oven to 350 degrees F (175 degrees C).
4. Cook and stir ground beef in a large skillet over medium heat until no longer pink and completely browned, 7 to 10 minutes; season with salt and black pepper. Stir cream of mushroom soup into the cooked ground beef; pour the mixture into a 9x13-inch baking dish. Layer tater tots evenly

over the ground beef mixture; top with Cheddar cheese.

5. Bake until tater tots are golden brown and hot, 30 to 45 minutes.